Hypertrophy Muscle Growth Guide for Beginners

Understanding the Benefits of Hypertrophy Muscle

By

Gregor Ezequiel

Table of Contents

CHAPTER 1 5

Introduction...5

1.1 Understanding Muscle
Hypertrophy.....................................6

1.2 Setting Realistic Expectations 8

CHAPTER 2 12

The Science Behind Muscle
Hypertrophy 12

2.1 Muscle Anatomy and Function 12

2.2 Mechanisms of Muscle Growth14

2.3 The Role of Nutrition in
Hypertrophy....................................16

CHAPTER 3 20

Designing Your Workout Program....20

3.1 Goal Setting...............................20

3.2 Choosing the Right Exercises...23

3.3 Structuring Your Training Split26

3.4 Repetitions, Sets, and Rest Periods 29

3.5 Progressive Overload 32

CHAPTER 4 35

Nutrition for Muscle Growth 35

4.1 The Importance of Protein 35

4.2 Carbohydrates and Fats for Energy 37

4.3 Caloric Surplus vs. Deficit 40

4.4 Meal Timing and Frequency 42

4.5 Supplements for Beginners 46

CHAPTER 5 49

Recovery and Rest 49

5.1 Sleep and Its Impact on Muscle Growth 49

5.2 The Role of Rest Days 51

5.3 Managing Muscle Soreness 54

CHAPTER 6 60

Tracking Progress 60

6.1 Importance of Tracking 60

6.2 Measuring Strength and Muscle Growth 63

6.3 Keeping a Workout Journal 67

CHAPTER 7 74

Common Mistakes to Avoid 74

7.1 Overtraining 74

7.2 Ignoring Proper Form 77

7.3 Neglecting Recovery 80

7.4 Focusing Solely on Isolation Exercises 83

CHAPTER 8 87

Staying Motivated 87

8.1 Setting Short and Long-Term Goals 87

8.2 Finding Support and Accountability 91

8.3 Celebrating Your Achievements 95

CHAPTER 1

Introduction

The journey into the world of muscle hypertrophy is an exciting and transformative one. For beginners, it represents a foray into the realm of physical fitness that promises not only enhanced strength and vitality but also a profound change in one's physical appearance. This introductory section serves as the portal to the world of muscle hypertrophy, with a dual purpose: to help you comprehend the essential concept of muscle hypertrophy and to set realistic expectations for the journey that lies ahead.

1.1 Understanding Muscle Hypertrophy

Muscle hypertrophy, in its simplest terms, refers to the process by which muscles grow in size and strength. It is the physiological response of the body to resistance training and a well-structured exercise program. At the microscopic level, muscle fibers undergo repair and growth in response to the stress placed upon them during resistance exercises. These exercises, which could include weightlifting, bodyweight exercises, or resistance bands, initiate a cascade of cellular and molecular events within the muscle tissues. These events involve the recruitment of more muscle fibers, an increase in the cross-sectional area of individual muscle fibers, and enhanced protein synthesis, ultimately resulting in larger and stronger muscles.

Understanding muscle hypertrophy involves recognizing that it's not a uniform process for everyone. Genetic factors, age, gender, and other individual characteristics can influence the rate and extent of muscle growth. Moreover, the type of exercises, training intensity, and nutrition play pivotal roles in the hypertrophy process. For beginners, this knowledge sets the foundation for crafting a tailored approach to muscle growth that aligns with their unique physiology and goals.

It's important to note that muscle hypertrophy is not just about aesthetics; it has significant implications for overall health and fitness. As muscles grow stronger, they enhance metabolic rate, making it easier to manage body weight and improve body composition. Additionally, increased muscle mass can lead to better posture, joint stability, and overall physical function, which contributes to a higher quality of life.

1.2 Setting Realistic Expectations

Setting realistic expectations is a crucial aspect of embarking on a journey towards muscle hypertrophy. While the idea of building a muscular physique may be alluring, it's essential to understand that achieving significant results takes time, dedication, and patience. The transformation from a beginner to a seasoned practitioner of muscle hypertrophy is not a sprint; it's a marathon.

Realistic expectations begin with acknowledging that progress is gradual. Gains in muscle size and strength occur over weeks and months, not days. For beginners, it's vital to embrace the concept of progressive overload, which involves consistently increasing the resistance or intensity of exercises to stimulate muscle growth. However, this doesn't mean that you'll witness massive changes after a few workouts. Rather, you'll experience incremental improvements that, over time, accumulate into substantial progress.

Another key aspect of setting realistic expectations is understanding that there will be obstacles and setbacks along the way. Plateaus, injuries, and periods of slower progress are not uncommon in the world of muscle hypertrophy. These should not be seen as failures but rather as opportunities for learning and adaptation. Staying committed and patient during such phases is critical to long-term success.

Furthermore, it's essential to realize that the rate of muscle growth is influenced by various factors, including genetics, age, and individual response to training. Some beginners may experience faster gains than others, but this should not deter anyone from pursuing their goals. Everyone's journey is unique, and it's crucial to focus on your own progress rather than comparing it to others.

understanding muscle hypertrophy and setting realistic expectations at the outset of your journey is the foundation for success in your pursuit of enhanced strength and physical transformation. By grasping the fundamental principles of muscle growth and approaching your goals with patience and dedication, you'll be well-prepared for the challenges and triumphs that lie ahead in your quest for muscle hypertrophy.

CHAPTER 2

The Science Behind Muscle Hypertrophy

2.1 Muscle Anatomy and Function

Before delving into the intricacies of muscle hypertrophy, it's essential to understand the basics of muscle anatomy and function. Muscles are the contractile tissues of the body responsible for generating force and facilitating movement. They are composed of muscle fibers, which are the individual cells that contract to create movement.

There are three main types of muscle in the human body: skeletal muscle, cardiac muscle, and smooth muscle. In the context of muscle hypertrophy, we primarily focus on skeletal muscle, which is the type of muscle responsible for voluntary movement. Skeletal muscles are attached to bones via tendons and work in pairs to move our limbs and maintain posture.

Muscle contraction is initiated by electrical signals from the nervous system. When you decide to lift a weight or perform any movement, your brain sends signals to your muscles, causing them to contract. This contraction shortens the muscle fibers and generates force, enabling you to perform various physical activities.

Muscle anatomy varies from one muscle group to another. Understanding the anatomy of the muscles you intend to target in your training program is crucial. It helps you select the appropriate exercises and training methods to stimulate hypertrophy in those specific muscle groups.

2.2 Mechanisms of Muscle Growth

The process of muscle hypertrophy is governed by several fundamental mechanisms. To trigger muscle growth, it's essential to subject your muscles to stress or resistance. When you engage in resistance training, such as weightlifting or bodyweight exercises, you create micro-tears in the muscle fibers. These micro-tears are a natural response to the mechanical stress placed on the muscles during exercise.

The body's response to these micro-tears involves a series of events, including muscle protein synthesis and satellite cell activation. Satellite cells are dormant cells located around muscle fibers, and when muscle damage occurs, they become activated to facilitate muscle repair and growth. Muscle protein synthesis is the process by which the body builds new proteins, which are used to repair and strengthen the muscle fibers.

As part of this repair and growth process, the muscle fibers increase in size and, with repeated training and adaptation, they become thicker and stronger. This adaptation is driven by the principle of progressive overload, which involves consistently increasing the resistance or intensity of your workouts. Over time, this adaptation results in noticeable gains in muscle size and strength.

2.3 The Role of Nutrition in Hypertrophy

Nutrition is a cornerstone of muscle hypertrophy. What you eat significantly impacts your body's ability to grow and repair muscle tissue. To support muscle growth effectively, you need to provide your body with the right nutrients. Here are some key components of nutrition in the context of hypertrophy:

- **Protein**: Protein is the building block of muscle tissue. Consuming an adequate amount of protein is crucial for muscle repair and growth. Amino acids, the building blocks of protein, are necessary for the synthesis of new muscle proteins.

- **Caloric Intake**: To gain muscle mass, you need to consume more calories than you burn, creating a caloric surplus. This provides your body with the energy required for muscle growth. However, it's essential to strike a balance and avoid excessive calorie consumption, which can lead to unwanted fat gain.

- **Macronutrients**: Carbohydrates and fats provide the energy needed for workouts and overall function. Carbohydrates are particularly important for high-intensity exercise, while fats are essential for hormone regulation and overall health.

- **Micronutrients**: Vitamins and minerals play a vital role in various physiological processes, including muscle function and repair. Ensuring you get an adequate intake of vitamins and minerals is essential for overall health and muscle growth.

- **Hydration**: Proper hydration is necessary for muscle function and recovery. Dehydration can lead to decreased exercise performance and hinder muscle growth.

Incorporating these nutritional principles into your diet, along with proper timing of meals and snacks, can significantly enhance the results of your muscle hypertrophy efforts. A well-balanced diet that supports your energy needs and provides the essential nutrients is a fundamental component of a successful muscle-building journey.

CHAPTER 3

Designing Your Workout Program

3.1 Goal Setting

Setting clear and achievable goals is the first step in designing an effective workout program for muscle hypertrophy. Your goals provide direction and motivation, helping you stay on track throughout your fitness journey. When setting your goals, consider the following:

- **Specificity**: Define your objectives clearly. Do you want to gain a certain amount of muscle mass, increase strength, improve endurance, or work on specific muscle groups? The

more specific your goals, the
easier it is to create a targeted
plan.

- **Measurability**: Ensure your
goals are measurable. For
example, if your aim is to
increase muscle mass, you can
set a goal to gain a certain
number of pounds or inches in
specific muscle groups.

- **Realism**: Be realistic about
what you can achieve. While
it's important to aim high,
setting unattainable goals can
lead to frustration. Consider
your current fitness level,
available time, and
commitment.

- **Timeframe**: Establish a
timeframe for your goals.
Having a deadline creates a

sense of urgency and helps you stay focused. However, make sure your timeline is realistic; substantial muscle growth takes time.

- **Long-Term vs. Short-Term Goals**: Distinguish between short-term and long-term goals. Short-term goals can help you stay motivated and track your progress, while long-term goals provide a broader vision for your fitness journey.

By setting well-defined and achievable goals, you'll have a clear sense of purpose, which will guide your exercise selection, training split, and overall workout program.

3.2 Choosing the Right Exercises

Selecting the right exercises is crucial for an effective muscle hypertrophy workout program. You should focus on exercises that target the specific muscle groups you want to develop. Here are some considerations when choosing exercises:

- **Compound vs. Isolation**: Compound exercises involve multiple muscle groups and joints, making them efficient for overall muscle growth. Examples include squats, deadlifts, and bench presses. Isolation exercises, on the other hand, target a single muscle group, such as bicep curls or leg extensions. A balanced program should include both compound and isolation exercises.

- **Variety**: To prevent plateaus and maintain motivation, incorporate a variety of exercises. This not only challenges your muscles in different ways but also keeps your workouts interesting.

- **Form and Technique**: Proper form and technique are paramount. Using correct form not only minimizes the risk of injury but also ensures that you're effectively targeting the intended muscle group.

- **Equipment Availability**: Consider the equipment you have access to, whether it's a fully equipped gym or limited home equipment. Your exercise selection should align with the equipment available to you.

- **Progressive Overload**: Choose exercises that allow for progressive overload. This means you can gradually increase the resistance or intensity of the exercise as you get stronger, which is essential for muscle growth.

- **Balanced Muscle Development**: Ensure that your exercise selection promotes balanced muscle development. Neglecting certain muscle groups can lead to imbalances and potentially cause injury.

3.3 Structuring Your Training Split

A training split refers to how you organize and distribute your workouts throughout the week. There are several training splits to choose from, and the one you select should align with your goals, schedule, and recovery capacity. Here are a few common training splits:

- **Full-Body Workouts**: In a full-body workout, you target all major muscle groups in a single session. This approach is great for beginners and those with limited time for exercise. It allows for frequent training of each muscle group, promoting balanced development.

- **Upper-Lower Split**: An upper-lower split involves dedicating one workout day to upper body exercises and another day to lower body exercises. This approach allows for more focused training of specific muscle groups and is often used by intermediate and advanced trainees.

- **Push-Pull-Legs (PPL) Split**: The PPL split separates workouts into push (chest, shoulders, triceps), pull (back, biceps), and legs. This approach offers a balanced training regimen and is popular among those seeking well-rounded muscle development.

- **Body-Part Split**: This split involves targeting specific muscle groups on different days. For example, you might have a day dedicated to chest, another for back, and so on. Body-part splits are common among bodybuilders and can allow for in-depth targeting of muscle groups.

The choice of training split should align with your goals and schedule. Additionally, it's crucial to include adequate rest and recovery days in your split to prevent overtraining and support muscle repair and growth. Your training split should also consider your level of experience, as more advanced trainees may benefit from higher training frequency for specific muscle groups.

3.4 Repetitions, Sets, and Rest Periods

The way you structure your repetitions (reps), sets, and rest periods in your workout program plays a significant role in achieving muscle hypertrophy. These variables determine the intensity and volume of your workouts. Here's a breakdown of each aspect:

- **Repetitions (Reps)**: Repetitions refer to the number of times you perform a specific exercise in one set. The number of reps you choose influences the training effect. In the context of hypertrophy, a common range is 6-12 reps per set. This range is often referred to as the "hypertrophy range" because it combines sufficient resistance to stimulate muscle growth while also allowing for an adequate number of repetitions.

- **Sets**: A set is a group of repetitions. For example, if you perform 10 squats, take a rest, and then perform another 10 squats, you've completed two sets of 10 reps each. The number of sets you perform determines the overall volume of your workout. Beginners often start with 3-4 sets per exercise, gradually increasing the volume as they progress.

- **Rest Periods**: The rest period between sets is crucial for recovery and performance. Shorter rest periods (30-60 seconds) tend to induce more metabolic stress and can be effective for muscle hypertrophy. Longer rest periods (2-3 minutes) allow for better strength recovery between sets and can be beneficial when using heavier weights. The choice of rest period depends on your goals and the intensity of your workout.

The specific combination of these variables can be adjusted to create different training effects. For example, you might choose to perform 3 sets of 10-12 reps with shorter rest periods to focus on muscle endurance and metabolic stress. Alternatively, you could opt for 4 sets of 6-8 reps with longer rest periods to emphasize strength development.

3.5 Progressive Overload

Progressive overload is a fundamental principle in muscle hypertrophy. It refers to the gradual increase in the resistance or intensity of your workouts over time. To promote muscle growth, your muscles need to be consistently challenged beyond their current capacity. Here's how progressive overload works:

- **Increasing Resistance**: The most common way to achieve progressive overload is by increasing the amount of weight you lift. This can be done by adding weight plates to a barbell, dumbbell, or using resistance bands, among other methods. Gradually lifting heavier weights forces your muscles to adapt and grow.

- **Increasing Repetitions or Sets**: You can also achieve progressive overload by increasing the number of repetitions or sets you perform. For example, if you started with 3 sets of 8 reps, you can aim to perform 3 sets of 10 reps in your next workout.

- **Improving Technique**: Bettering your exercise technique can also be a form of progressive overload. As your form becomes more precise and efficient, you can effectively target the intended muscle groups and stimulate more muscle fibers.

- **Varying Exercises**: Changing or adding exercises to your routine can provide a different stimulus for muscle growth.

This variety can help prevent plateaus and promote continuous progress.

- **Reducing Rest Periods**: Shortening rest periods between sets can increase the intensity of your workouts and create a form of progressive overload, especially when focusing on metabolic stress and endurance.

Effective progressive overload requires tracking your progress, whether through a workout journal or using fitness apps. By systematically and consistently increasing the demands on your muscles, you encourage them to adapt and grow, driving ongoing muscle hypertrophy over time. Remember that progressive overload is a gradual process, and patience is key to its success.

CHAPTER 4

Nutrition for Muscle Growth

4.1 The Importance of Protein

Protein is a cornerstone of nutrition for muscle growth, and its significance cannot be overstated. It plays several critical roles in the muscle hypertrophy process:

- **Muscle Repair and Growth**: Protein provides the essential building blocks, called amino acids, required for the repair and growth of muscle tissue. When you engage in resistance training, you create micro-tears in your muscle fibers. Protein aids in the repair and regeneration of these fibers, leading to muscle growth and increased strength.

- **Hormone Production**: Several hormones are involved in muscle growth, including insulin, testosterone, and growth hormone. Protein intake influences the production and regulation of these hormones, further supporting muscle development.

- **Satiety and Weight Management**: Protein has a high satiety value, meaning it helps you feel full and satisfied. This can be beneficial for managing caloric intake and body weight, as it reduces the likelihood of overeating.

For individuals aiming to maximize muscle hypertrophy, it's recommended to consume an adequate amount of protein from various sources, including lean meats, poultry, fish, dairy products, eggs, and plant-based options like legumes and tofu. The specific protein requirements can vary depending on factors like age, gender, activity level, and goals, but a general guideline is to aim for around 1.2 to 2.2 grams of protein per kilogram of body weight per day. Consuming protein both before and after workouts can support muscle protein synthesis and repair.

4.2 Carbohydrates and Fats for Energy

Carbohydrates and fats are essential macronutrients that provide the energy required for workouts and daily activities. They are valuable for muscle growth in several ways:

- **Energy Source**: Carbohydrates are the body's primary energy source, particularly during high-intensity exercise. Fats also serve as an energy source during low to moderate-intensity activities and are crucial for overall health.

- **Hormone Regulation**: Both carbohydrates and fats play roles in hormone regulation, including insulin, which influences nutrient uptake by muscle cells. Stable hormone levels are important for muscle growth.

- **Caloric Support**: Carbohydrates and fats

contribute to your overall
caloric intake. To create a
caloric surplus (discussed in the
next section), you need an
adequate amount of these
macronutrients to support
muscle growth.

Balancing your carbohydrate and fat
intake depends on your individual
needs, activity level, and dietary
preferences. Generally, carbohydrates
should make up a significant portion
of your daily caloric intake,
particularly on workout days when
energy demands are higher. Healthy
sources of carbohydrates include
whole grains, fruits, vegetables, and
legumes. Fats, which are important
for overall health, can be sourced
from nuts, seeds, avocados, and
healthy oils.

4.3 Caloric Surplus vs. Deficit

The balance between caloric intake and expenditure is a crucial factor in muscle growth. It determines whether you are in a caloric surplus, maintenance, or deficit. Understanding this balance is essential:

- **Caloric Surplus**: To promote muscle growth, you typically need to be in a caloric surplus, which means you are consuming more calories than you burn. The surplus provides the extra energy needed for muscle repair and growth. However, it's essential to maintain a controlled surplus, as excessive caloric intake can lead to unwanted fat gain. A moderate surplus, typically

250-500 calories above
maintenance, is often
recommended for muscle
building.

- **Maintenance**: Maintaining a
stable caloric balance (calories
in equal to calories out) is ideal
for those who wish to maintain
their current body weight and
composition without significant
changes.

- **Caloric Deficit**: A caloric
deficit occurs when you
consume fewer calories than
you burn. This is typically
associated with weight loss and
fat reduction, not muscle
growth. However, there are
strategies to minimize muscle
loss during a cutting phase,
such as adequate protein intake
and resistance training.

The specific caloric balance that's right for you depends on your goals. If muscle hypertrophy is your primary objective, then a controlled caloric surplus combined with a well-structured exercise program is key. On the other hand, if fat loss is also a goal, you may use periods of caloric surplus to promote muscle growth alternated with periods of caloric deficit to reduce body fat. Balancing your macronutrients and monitoring your caloric intake is vital to ensure you are fueling your body optimally for muscle growth.

4.4 Meal Timing and Frequency

Meal timing and frequency can influence your muscle growth and overall performance. While these factors are important, it's essential to understand that individual preferences and schedules can greatly impact your approach. Here are some key considerations:

- **Pre-Workout Nutrition**: Consuming a balanced meal or snack before your workout provides the energy needed for optimal performance. Including carbohydrates for energy and protein for muscle support is a good practice. Timing-wise, aim to eat 1-2 hours before exercise to allow for digestion.

- **Post-Workout Nutrition**: After your workout, your body is primed for nutrient absorption and muscle recovery. A post-workout meal or protein shake rich in carbohydrates and protein can help replenish glycogen stores and support muscle protein synthesis. Consuming this meal within 30-60 minutes after exercise is often recommended, but the anabolic window is not as narrow as previously believed, and overall daily nutrition is more important.

- **Meal Frequency**: The number of meals you consume daily can vary based on your preferences and lifestyle. Some people prefer three square meals a day, while others thrive with smaller, more frequent meals. Research shows that meal frequency may not significantly impact muscle growth as long as you meet your daily macronutrient and caloric needs.

- **Balanced Nutrition**: Regardless of meal timing and frequency, focus on balanced nutrition. Ensure each meal contains a combination of protein, carbohydrates, and healthy fats to support overall health and muscle growth.

- **Hydration**: Staying hydrated is critical for muscle function and recovery. Drink water throughout the day and consider electrolyte-rich beverages if you engage in intense workouts that lead to significant sweat loss.

- **Individual Adaptation**: Everyone's body reacts differently to meal timing and frequency. It's important to experiment and find a routine that suits your needs, energy levels, and workout performance.

4.5 Supplements for Beginners

While whole foods should be the foundation of your nutrition plan, some supplements may complement your diet and support your muscle-building efforts. Here are a few supplements that beginners may consider:

- **Protein Supplements**: Protein powders, such as whey protein or plant-based alternatives, can help you meet your daily protein requirements more conveniently. They are particularly useful for post-workout nutrition and when whole food sources of protein are unavailable.

- **Creatine**: Creatine is a naturally occurring compound found in small amounts in some foods and produced by the body. It's one of the most researched and effective supplements for increasing strength and promoting muscle growth. Creatine monohydrate is a common and cost-effective form.

- **Branched-Chain Amino Acids (BCAAs)**: BCAAs are amino acids that can be consumed as supplements. They may support muscle protein synthesis, reduce muscle soreness, and provide energy during workouts. However, if you consume enough protein from your diet, BCAAs may not be necessary.

- **Multivitamins**: A high-quality multivitamin can help ensure you receive essential vitamins and minerals for overall health. However, if your diet is well-balanced, you may not need a multivitamin.

It's important to note that supplements should be used to complement a well-rounded diet, not as a replacement for whole foods. If you're considering adding supplements to your regimen, consult with a healthcare professional or registered dietitian to determine what may be appropriate for your specific needs. Additionally, always choose reputable brands and products to ensure quality and safety.

CHAPTER 5

Recovery and Rest

5.1 Sleep and Its Impact on Muscle Growth

Sleep is an often underestimated but vital component of muscle growth and overall health. It's during sleep that your body goes through various restorative processes, many of which directly affect muscle growth. Here's how sleep impacts muscle growth:

- **Muscle Recovery**: During deep sleep, your body engages in muscle repair and growth. This is when it synthesizes new proteins, repairs damaged muscle fibers, and replenishes glycogen stores, all crucial for hypertrophy.

- **Hormone Regulation**: Sleep plays a key role in regulating hormones that are critical for muscle growth, such as growth hormone and testosterone. Insufficient sleep can disrupt hormonal balance, potentially hindering muscle development.

- **Energy Restoration**: Adequate sleep ensures that your energy levels are replenished for your workouts. Sleep-deprived individuals often experience reduced physical and mental performance, which can impede effective training.

To support muscle growth, aim for 7-9 hours of quality sleep each night. Establish a consistent sleep schedule, create a sleep-conducive environment (cool, dark, and quiet), and limit caffeine and electronic device use close to bedtime. Prioritizing good sleep hygiene is an investment in your muscle-building goals.

5.2 The Role of Rest Days

Rest days are an integral part of a well-structured workout program, and they are often underestimated in their importance for muscle growth. Here's why rest days matter:

- **Muscle Recovery**: During resistance training, your muscles experience micro-tears. Rest days allow your body to repair and rebuild these muscle fibers, contributing to muscle growth and enhanced strength.

- **Prevention of Overtraining**: Overtraining, a state of excessive exercise without adequate recovery, can lead to decreased performance, increased risk of injury, and hindered muscle growth. Rest days provide your body with the opportunity to recover, reducing the risk of overtraining.

- **Mental Recovery**: Rest days not only benefit your body but also your mind. They can help you avoid burnout and maintain motivation for consistent training in the long term.

- **Preventing Plateaus**: Continuous, intense training without rest can lead to performance plateaus. Incorporating rest days and varying workout intensity can help break through plateaus and stimulate further progress.

The frequency of rest days can vary depending on your individual needs, training intensity, and experience level. Beginners may benefit from 2-3 rest days per week, while more advanced individuals might have fewer rest days or employ active recovery techniques like yoga or light cardio on rest days. The key is to listen to your body and recognize when it needs rest and recovery.

Rest days don't mean you have to be entirely sedentary. Active recovery, such as low-intensity activities or mobility work, can aid in muscle recovery without adding significant stress to your body. Ultimately, the right balance between training and rest is crucial for consistent muscle growth and overall well-being.

5.3 Managing Muscle Soreness

Muscle soreness, often referred to as delayed onset muscle soreness (DOMS), is a common sensation experienced after intense or unfamiliar exercise. While it can be uncomfortable, it's a normal part of the muscle-building process. Here's how to manage and alleviate muscle soreness:

- **Proper Warm-Up and Cool-Down**: Before starting your workout, ensure you engage in a proper warm-up to increase blood flow and prepare your muscles for exercise. After your

workout, perform a cool-down
routine to gradually reduce
your heart rate and prevent
blood pooling in your muscles.
This can help minimize post-
workout soreness.

- **Hydration**: Staying well-
  hydrated is essential for muscle
  function and recovery.
  Dehydration can exacerbate
  muscle soreness, so be sure to
  drink enough water throughout
  the day.

- **Nutrition**: Consuming a
  balanced diet with adequate
  protein, carbohydrates, and
  healthy fats is important for
  muscle recovery. Proper
  nutrition supports the repair and
  growth of muscle tissue.

- **Stretching**: Incorporating gentle stretching exercises, such as static or dynamic stretching, can help improve flexibility and reduce muscle tension. Stretching may provide relief from muscle soreness.

- **Foam Rolling**: Using a foam roller or other self-massage tools can help release muscle tension and alleviate soreness. Foam rolling is often used for self-myofascial release (SMR) to target trigger points in the muscles.

- **Rest and Recovery**: Adequate rest and recovery days are crucial. Sore muscles need time to repair and grow. Give your body the opportunity to heal by incorporating rest days into your training schedule.

- **Over-the-Counter Pain Relief**: Non-prescription pain relief options, such as over-the-counter nonsteroidal anti-inflammatory drugs (NSAIDs) like ibuprofen, can provide temporary relief from muscle soreness. However, they should be used sparingly and as directed.

- **Massage**: Professional massages can help reduce muscle tension and soreness. A massage therapist can target specific muscle groups and apply techniques to alleviate discomfort.

- **Gradual Progression**: When increasing the intensity or volume of your workouts, do so gradually. This can help prevent excessive muscle soreness due to rapid changes in training stimulus.

- **Active Recovery**: Engaging in light, low-impact activities, such as walking or swimming, on rest days or after intense workouts can help promote blood flow and ease muscle soreness.

muscle soreness is typically at its peak 24-48 hours after a workout and tends to subside within a few days. If soreness persists or becomes severe, it may indicate an injury, and you should seek professional medical advice.

some degree of muscle soreness is normal and can be a sign of productive training. As your body adapts to your exercise routine, soreness tends to decrease over time.

Embrace it as a sign of progress in
your muscle-building journey.

CHAPTER 6

Tracking Progress

6.1 Importance of Tracking

Tracking your progress is a crucial aspect of a successful muscle-building journey. It provides several benefits, helping you stay motivated, make informed decisions, and achieve your goals effectively. Here's why tracking is essential:

- **Motivation**: Tracking your progress allows you to see how far you've come. It can be highly motivating to witness improvements in strength, muscle size, and overall fitness. These visible gains can

encourage you to stick with
your program and continue
working toward your goals.

- **Goal Assessment**: Regularly
  tracking your progress enables
  you to assess whether you're on
  track to achieve your goals. If
  you're not making the desired
  progress, you can adjust your
  workout routine, nutrition, or
  other factors accordingly.

- **Identifying Plateaus**: Plateaus,
  where progress slows or stops,
  are a common challenge in
  muscle building. By tracking
  your progress, you can identify
  these plateaus and make
  necessary adjustments to break
  through them.

- **Objective Feedback**: Tracking
  provides objective feedback on

your performance. It allows you to see which exercises are effective, which need improvement, and where you may be falling short in terms of nutrition, rest, or other factors.

- **Goal Setting**: Tracking helps you set realistic and achievable goals. It provides a baseline against which you can measure your future progress. By setting specific, measurable, and time-bound goals, you can create a roadmap for your journey.

- **Accountability**: When you track your progress, you become more accountable for your actions. Knowing that you'll record your results can encourage you to stay consistent with your training and nutrition plan.

- **Preventing Injury**: Monitoring your progress helps you avoid overtraining and reduces the risk of injury. If you notice signs of overtraining, you can adjust your training volume or intensity to protect your health.

6.2 Measuring Strength and Muscle Growth

To track your muscle-building progress effectively, you'll want to use various methods to measure both strength and muscle growth. Here are some ways to do so:

- **Strength Measurements**: Measuring strength is a clear indicator of muscle development because, as your muscles grow, they typically become stronger. You can track strength through various means:

- **One-Rep Max (1RM)**: This is the maximum weight you can lift for a single repetition of a given exercise. Tracking your 1RM over time can help you see strength improvements.

- **Repetition Max (RM)**: This involves measuring the maximum weight you can lift for a specific number of repetitions. For example, your 5RM is the heaviest weight you can lift for 5 reps. This method is useful for tracking progress in lower-repetition strength training programs.

- **Progressive Overload**: By consistently increasing the weight or resistance used in your exercises over time, you can monitor your strength gains. If you're lifting heavier weights or performing more repetitions with a given weight, you're making progress.

- **Muscle Measurements**: Tracking muscle size is another key aspect of monitoring your progress. You can measure muscle growth by:

  - **Circumference Measurements**: Use a

tape measure to measure the circumference of specific muscle groups, such as your biceps, chest, thighs, or calves. Record these measurements over time to track growth.

- **Visual Assessment**: Regularly taking photos of your physique under consistent conditions and lighting can help you visually assess changes in muscle size and definition.

- **Body Composition Analysis**: Utilizing body composition measurement tools like skinfold calipers, bioelectrical impedance scales, or DEXA scans can provide insights into changes in muscle and fat mass.

Progress in muscle building can sometimes be slow and gradual. Tracking your strength and muscle size over an extended period, rather than just a few weeks, will provide a more accurate reflection of your accomplishments. Be patient, stay consistent, and use tracking as a tool to stay motivated and informed on your journey to muscle growth.

6.3 Keeping a Workout Journal

Keeping a workout journal is an effective and practical way to track your progress, stay organized, and optimize your muscle-building journey. Here's why and how to maintain a workout journal:

Why Keep a Workout Journal:

1. **Accountability**: A workout journal holds you accountable. When you record your workouts, you're more likely to stick to your training program and stay consistent.

2. **Progress Tracking**: It allows you to monitor your progress over time. You can see how your strength, endurance, and muscle size are improving, helping you make informed decisions about your training.

3. **Identifying Patterns**: By reviewing your journal, you can identify patterns in your performance. For example, you

might notice that you're consistently stronger on certain days or with specific exercises. This information can help you plan your workouts more effectively.

4. **Goal Setting**: A workout journal is a valuable tool for setting and achieving goals. You can establish specific targets for weight lifted, repetitions, or other performance markers and track your journey toward those goals.

5. **Nutrition and Recovery**: You can use your journal to log information about your nutrition, sleep, and recovery. This provides a comprehensive view of your health and can

help you identify factors that affect your training.

How to Keep a Workout Journal:

1. **Select a Journal**: Choose a physical notebook or use a digital app or spreadsheet to record your workouts. There are many workout journal apps available for smartphones.

2. **Plan Your Workouts**: Before each training session, plan your workout. Write down the exercises, sets, repetitions, and weights you intend to use. Having a plan will keep you focused and organized.

3. **Record Each Workout**: During your workout, record your actual performance. Include the date, exercises, sets, reps, and weights lifted. You

can also note how the workout felt and any adjustments you made on the fly.

4. **Review and Analyze**: Periodically review your journal to track your progress. Look for trends, improvements, or areas where you need to make changes. Use this information to adjust your program as necessary.

5. **Set Goals**: Based on your progress, set realistic short-term and long-term goals. These can be related to strength, muscle size, or any other aspect of your training.

6. **Document Nutrition and Recovery**: Consider logging your daily nutrition, including macronutrient intake, meal

timing, and hydration. Additionally, record details about your sleep and recovery practices to assess their impact on your performance.

7. **Stay Consistent**: Make journaling a consistent habit. Record every workout, even if it feels routine. Over time, this comprehensive record will become a valuable resource.

8. **Use Technology**: If you prefer digital methods, explore workout journal apps and online tools. These often come with features like progress tracking, goal setting, and even video demonstrations of exercises.

Your workout journal is a personal tool, and you can customize it to your needs. The goal is to make it as user-friendly and informative as possible. Whether you're a beginner or an experienced athlete, a workout journal can help you maximize your muscle-building efforts and fine-tune your training program for optimal results.

CHAPTER 7

Common Mistakes to Avoid

7.1 Overtraining

Overtraining is a common mistake that can hinder your muscle-building progress and even lead to physical and mental burnout. Overtraining occurs when you don't allow your body enough time to recover between workouts, and it can manifest in various ways, including decreased performance, muscle soreness, and even increased risk of injury. Here's how to avoid overtraining:

- **Implement Rest Days**: Ensure you incorporate rest days into your training schedule. These rest days allow your muscles to recover and repair. The frequency of rest days can vary depending on your training program, but it's essential to give your body the time it needs to recuperate.

- **Listen to Your Body**: Pay attention to signs of overtraining, such as chronic fatigue, persistent soreness, reduced strength, or a drop in motivation. If you notice these symptoms, consider adjusting your workout intensity or taking additional rest days.

- **Vary Your Routine**: Overtraining can result from doing the same exercises or routines too frequently. Incorporate variety into your workouts to avoid overloading specific muscle groups and joints. This can also prevent mental burnout.

- **Get Adequate Sleep**: As discussed earlier, sleep is essential for recovery. Prioritize quality sleep to help your body recuperate from intense workouts and reduce the risk of overtraining.

- **Nutrition Matters**: Ensure you're eating a balanced diet with sufficient nutrients to support your training. Undernourishment can contribute to overtraining, so fuel your body appropriately.

- **Progressive Overload**: As mentioned in a previous section, progressive overload is vital for muscle growth.

However, avoid the temptation to increase weights or intensity too rapidly. Gradual progression is key to avoiding overtraining.

7.2 Ignoring Proper Form

Proper form is essential for safety, effectiveness, and muscle growth. Ignoring it can lead to injuries and suboptimal results. Here's how to avoid common form mistakes:

- **Learn Proper Technique**: Before you begin any exercise, make sure you understand the correct form. This might involve working with a qualified trainer or watching instructional videos. Proper technique ensures you're targeting the right muscle groups and reducing the risk of injury.

- **Focus on Control**: Avoid using momentum to lift weights. Instead, concentrate on controlled movements. This not only maximizes muscle engagement but also minimizes the risk of accidents.

- **Use a Mirror**: Exercising in front of a mirror can help you monitor your form. This is especially helpful for exercises where form is crucial, such as squats and deadlifts.

- **Start with Light Weights**: When learning a new exercise or refining your form, begin with lighter weights. As you become more confident and comfortable, gradually increase the weight.

- **Mind-Muscle Connection**: Develop a mind-muscle connection by concentrating on the muscle you're working during each exercise. This mental focus can help ensure you're engaging the right muscles and using proper form.

- **Warm Up Properly**: A proper warm-up is essential to prepare your body for exercise and prevent injuries. Incorporate dynamic stretching and mobility exercises in your warm-up routine.

- **Seek Feedback**: If you're uncertain about your form, don't hesitate to ask for feedback from a knowledgeable friend, trainer, or use mirrors and video recordings to evaluate your technique.

Proper form not only maximizes the benefits of your workouts but also minimizes the risk of injury. It's worth taking the time to learn and practice good form from the outset and to continually monitor and refine your technique as you progress in your muscle-building journey.

7.3 Neglecting Recovery

Neglecting recovery is a common mistake that can impede muscle growth and increase the risk of overtraining and injury. Recovery is an essential part of the muscle-building process, and it goes beyond rest days. Here's how to avoid neglecting recovery:

- **Prioritize Sleep**: Adequate sleep is crucial for muscle recovery. Aim for 7-9 hours of quality sleep each night to allow your body to repair and grow.

- **Nutrition**: Proper nutrition plays a key role in recovery. Ensure you're consuming enough calories, macronutrients (protein, carbohydrates, and fats), and micronutrients to support your workouts and muscle growth.

- **Hydration**: Stay well-hydrated to support muscle function and recovery. Dehydration can lead to muscle cramps and decreased performance.

- **Active Recovery**: On rest days, consider engaging in light, low-impact activities like walking, swimming, or gentle stretching. These activities can promote blood flow and aid in recovery without causing additional stress.

- **Foam Rolling and Mobility**: Incorporate foam rolling and mobility exercises into your routine to alleviate muscle tension and improve flexibility. These practices can reduce the risk of injury and enhance recovery.

- **Manage Stress**: High stress levels can hinder recovery. Incorporate stress-reduction techniques, such as meditation, deep breathing, or yoga, into your routine.

- **Listen to Your Body**: Pay attention to how your body feels. If you're feeling fatigued, excessively sore, or unmotivated, it may be a sign that you need more recovery time.

- **Avoid Overtraining**: As mentioned earlier, overtraining can lead to decreased performance and hinder recovery. Be mindful of your training volume and intensity, and don't push your body beyond its limits.

7.4 Focusing Solely on Isolation Exercises

While isolation exercises have their place in a muscle-building program, focusing solely on them can be a mistake. Isolation exercises target specific muscle groups, but they often involve less weight and can be less efficient for overall muscle development. Here's how to avoid the pitfall of solely focusing on isolation exercises:

- **Incorporate Compound Exercises**: Compound exercises, such as squats, deadlifts, bench presses, and pull-ups, engage multiple muscle groups simultaneously. They allow you to lift heavier weights and stimulate more muscle fibers, contributing to greater overall muscle growth.

- **Balanced Training**: A balanced training program should include both isolation and compound exercises.

Isolation exercises can be useful for targeting specific muscles or addressing muscle imbalances, while compound exercises provide a foundation for strength and overall muscle development.

- **Variation**: Don't stick to the same exercises repeatedly. Incorporate a variety of compound and isolation exercises to challenge your muscles from different angles and promote well-rounded development.

- **Functional Strength**: Compound exercises tend to have a higher carryover to functional strength, making them valuable not only for muscle growth but also for improved performance in everyday activities.

- **Efficiency**: Compound exercises often require less time to complete a full-body workout. This can be particularly beneficial if you have limited time to spend at the gym.

The most effective muscle-building programs usually include a combination of compound and isolation exercises. The key is to strike a balance that suits your goals and individual needs. Compound exercises should form the foundation of your routine, while isolation exercises can be strategically incorporated to target specific muscle groups or address weaknesses.

CHAPTER 8

Staying Motivated

8.1 Setting Short and Long-Term Goals

Setting clear and achievable goals is a powerful motivator for your muscle-building journey. Goals give you direction and purpose, helping you stay on track and measure your progress. Here's how to set short and long-term goals:

Short-Term Goals:

1. **Specific Objectives**: Define clear and specific short-term goals. For example, aim to increase your bench press weight by 10 pounds in the next

two months or perform three sets of 10 pull-ups with proper form.

2. **Realistic Expectations**: Ensure your short-term goals are realistic and attainable within a relatively short time frame. Setting unattainable goals can be demotivating.

3. **Measurable Outcomes**: Your goals should have measurable outcomes. Use numbers and benchmarks to track your progress. This allows you to celebrate small victories along the way.

4. **Time Frame**: Set a time frame for your short-term goals. This creates a sense of urgency and commitment. For example, aim

to achieve your goal in four
weeks or three months.

5. **Relevance to Long-Term
   Goals**: Ensure that your short-
   term goals align with your
   long-term objectives. They
   should be stepping stones
   toward your larger aspirations.

Long-Term Goals:

1. **Big Picture Vision**: Long-term
   goals should reflect your
   ultimate vision for muscle
   growth and fitness. They may
   include achieving a certain
   level of strength, attaining a
   specific physique, or
   completing a fitness-related
   accomplishment (e.g., a
   marathon or bodybuilding
   competition).

2. **Break It Down**: Break down your long-term goals into smaller, manageable steps. These mini-goals become your short-term objectives.

3. **Maintain Flexibility**: Long-term goals should be adaptable. As you progress, you may need to adjust them based on your changing capabilities and circumstances.

4. **Visualize Success**: Create a mental image of what achieving your long-term goals looks like. Visualization can be a potent motivator.

5. **Stay Committed**: Long-term goals require patience and persistence. Keep your long-term vision in mind when faced with challenges or plateaus.

Regularly review and adjust your goals as you progress. This allows you to stay motivated and maintain a sense of purpose in your muscle-building journey.

8.2 Finding Support and Accountability

Building muscle and staying motivated is often easier with the support of others and a system of accountability. Here's how to find support and accountability:

1. **Training Partners**: Consider finding a workout partner or training buddy. Having someone to exercise with can provide motivation, friendly competition, and companionship. You can spot

each other during weightlifting, share workout routines, and help each other stay on track.

2. **Online Communities**: There are numerous online fitness communities, forums, and social media groups where you can connect with like-minded individuals. These platforms offer a wealth of information, motivation, and a sense of belonging.

3. **Fitness Apps**: Use fitness apps or tracking tools that allow you to share your progress with friends or fellow users. Some apps offer social features to create challenges and compete with others.

4. **Personal Trainer or Coach**: Hiring a personal trainer or

coach can provide expert guidance, motivation, and accountability. They can design tailored workouts, track your progress, and keep you on target.

5. **Accountability Partner**: Partner with a friend or family member who shares similar fitness goals. Share your progress regularly, hold each other accountable, and celebrate each other's successes.

6. **Join a Fitness Class or Group**: Participating in group fitness classes or sports leagues can be a fun way to stay motivated. The camaraderie and structure of classes or group activities can boost your commitment.

7. **Set Public Goals**: Announce your fitness goals to your social circle. When others are aware of your objectives, you may feel more motivated to achieve them to avoid the embarrassment of failure.

8. **Keep a Workout Journal**: As discussed earlier, a workout journal can serve as an accountability tool. Sharing your progress with a friend or trainer can help you stay on track.

Different people find motivation and accountability through various methods. Experiment with different strategies to find what works best for you. Combining social support with personal motivation can be a powerful combination to keep you committed to your muscle-building goals.

8.3 Celebrating Your Achievements

Celebrating your achievements, whether big or small, is a crucial aspect of staying motivated in your muscle-building journey. Recognizing your progress and milestones can boost your morale, maintain your commitment, and make the entire process more enjoyable. Here's how to celebrate your achievements:

1. Set Milestones: Break your long-term and short-term goals into smaller, measurable milestones. These milestones serve as checkpoints to assess your progress. When you reach a milestone, take a moment to celebrate.

2. Acknowledge the Effort: Recognize the hard work and dedication you've put into your workouts and nutrition. Your effort deserves acknowledgment, so don't be too modest to celebrate it.

3. Reward Yourself: Treat yourself to a reward when you achieve a significant goal. Rewards can be non-food related, like a new piece of fitness equipment, workout gear, or a relaxing spa day. Choose rewards that align with your fitness goals and values.

4. Share Your Success: Share your achievements with your support network, whether it's friends, family, or an online fitness community. Their encouragement and congratulations can be motivating and satisfying.

5. Document Your Progress: Keep a visual record of your achievements. Take before and after photos, track your strength gains, and measure changes in your physique. Comparing these visual records over time can be incredibly rewarding.

6. Reflect on the Journey: Take a moment to reflect on how far you've come. Consider the obstacles you've overcome and the improvements you've made. This reflection can help you appreciate the journey itself, not just the destination.

7. Use Positive Self-Talk: Cultivate a positive mindset by acknowledging your accomplishments. Instead of downplaying your successes, be your own biggest cheerleader and affirm your capabilities.

8. Set New Goals: After celebrating an achievement, set new goals to keep your motivation high. Having a fresh challenge on the horizon can maintain your enthusiasm for fitness.

9. Share Your Knowledge: If you've achieved something remarkable, consider sharing your knowledge and experience with others. This can be a source of fulfillment and motivation.

10. Celebrate Every Step: Don't limit your celebrations to major milestones. Acknowledge and appreciate even the small victories along the way. Whether it's lifting a slightly heavier weight or maintaining a consistent workout routine, these steps deserve recognition.

Celebrating your achievements is not only enjoyable but also important for sustaining your motivation in the long term. It reinforces the idea that your hard work pays off and can inspire you to continue pursuing your fitness goals with enthusiasm and determination.